Aging is a Treatable Disease
By Walter Parks
Kindle Edition

Copyright 2011 - 2015
UnKnownTruths
Publishing Company

All rights reserved. No part of this book may be used or reproduced in any manner whatsoever without written permission except in the case of brief quotations embodied in critical articles or reviews. For information please address the Publisher:
UnKnownTruths
Publishing Company
8815 Conroy Windermere Rd. Ste 190
Orlando, FL 32835
This book is also available in print.
My Website

This eBook is licensed for your personal enjoyment only. This eBook may not be re-sold or given away to other people. If you would like to share this book with another person, please purchase an additional copy for each recipient. If you're reading this book and did not purchase it, or it was not purchased for your use only, then please return to Smashwords.com and purchase your own copy. Thank you for respecting the hard work of this author.

Contents

Natural species are the library from which genetic engineers can work.
Thomas E. Lovejoy

"It is our duty, my young friends, to resist old age;

To compensate for its defects by a watchful care;

To fight against it as we would fight against disease;

To adopt a regimen of health; to practice moderate exercise;

And to take just enough food and drink to restore our strength;

And not to overburden it.

Cicero
106-43 BC

"The overall deterioration of the body that comes with growing old is not inevitable."

Dr. Rudman
After His Tests
June 1989

Acknowledgements

A great deal of the research for writing this book was accomplished with the Internet. Unfortunately most of the information found on the Internet is significantly biased. Everyone is trying to sell something. Some of the bias can be evident by comparing the information from the various competitors. But even when you begin to understand the biases you have to dig much deeper to get to the truth.

And lots of the time there is no obvious truth. More research, more digging in search of the truth is required.

Finally you get to the "best truth available". And that is what I have presented in this book.

I am deeply grateful to the many contributors to information on the Internet and to the wizards at Google for providing me the insight to the previously unknown truths presented in this book.

I thank them all.

Preface

Medical science and the unraveling of the human genome have, and are, providing us with great insights into how we work and how we are susceptible to diseases and the aging process.

Our new understandings now allow us to significantly increase our healthy longevity. And when we take advantages of these new findings we make ourselves available to take advantages of the even newer technologies being developed.

So if you want to increase your chances of living a long and healthy life you need to learn about what you can do. It is not very hard. You do not have to go to the extremes to get great benefits.

But you do need to learn and take action.

Review

Great Overview of Aging and How to Slow it Down!

⭐⭐⭐⭐⭐ By Brian S. Shore on March 18, 2013

This book first gives an overview as to what causes aging and then proceeds to describe several treatments available to slow down or reverse the effects of aging: from direct supplementation of HGH and other hormones by injection, to the much safer and less-expensive "Hormone Precursor Therapy"–using oral supplementation of various herbs, amino acids, foods and other substances to raise one's own levels of hormones naturally. The author also describes other treatments such as calorie restriction therapy, gene therapy, telomerase treatment, stress relief therapy, as well as some more futuristic possibilities. The short chapters are easy to read, and the broad range of treatments described makes this a book worthy of reading by anyone considering an anti-aging program.

Summary

"Over half the baby boomers here in America are going to see their hundredth birthday and beyond in excellent health. We're looking at life spans for the baby boomers and the generation after the baby boomers of 120 to 150 years of age." Dr. Ronald Klatz
American Academy
Of Anti-Aging

The overall deterioration of the body that comes with growing old is not inevitable.

Aging is a treatable disease.

I had a heart attack 14 years ago and another 8 years ago, and yet I live.

I had several TIAs (mini-strokes) 15 years ago and lost my memory. I have it back.

I had prostate cancer yet I am cured.

I had cataracts in both eyes yet I now see perfectly.

I had glaucoma yet I suffer no adverse consequences.

I was 70 pounds overweight yet my weight is now almost normal.

I looked 20 years older than my actual age, yet I now look 15 years younger than my actual age.

I am 75 and believe I will live pass 100.

There are actions you can take today to dramatically improve your health and longevity.

The causes of aging are finally being understood.

Dr. Rudman ran a series of tests on aging people and demonstrated that the effects of aging could be slowed and even reversed. He concluded:

"The overall deterioration of the body that comes with growing old is not inevitable."

Tens of millions die from age-related conditions each and every year. That is because they think that it is natural to get old and die. They do not know about, or do not take advantage of, the

7

programs that can already slow the processes and effects of degenerative aging.

America, and indeed the world, is aging. As the Baby Boomers retire over the next several years they will significantly change society. Their diseases that come with aging will drastically affect the health care industry. But you can do something about it.

Aging Is A Treatable Disease.

You need to learn what you can do today to make sure that you live long enough to take advantage of all the future medical innovations now in the works.

You have choices of what you can do:

Understand and put into practice a basic, proven anti-aging program specifically tailored to you. The future of medicine is in personal tailoring.

Understand the severity of stress and Practice Stress Therapy.

Understand and consider personally tailored Hormone Replacement Therapy (HRT), which has proven very effective but that may be risky.

Understand and consider personally tailored Hormone Precursor Therapy (HPT), which has proven effective but less so than HRT. A few also believe it may be somewhat risky since it has not had a long history.

Understand and consider the Calorie Restriction Program which can be effective but is far too uncomfortable for almost all people wishing to lead a normal life.

Understand and consider applying for Telomerase Therapy when is becomes available.

Understand and consider, if it applies to you, Gene Replacement Therapy.

Understand and participate in one or more of the as yet unproven "beta" programs resulting from the newly evolving technologies, when they become available.

Develop your own Personally Tailored Program that includes your selections from various combinations of all of the above. This will be your "full life plan".

I describe each of these in the following chapters. Hopefully I have included enough information to give you a good introduction to aging and to what you can do to increase your healthy longevity.

I am working with a group of experts to provide additional details and interactive Internet tools that will eventually be available to give you additional help to:

Live Healthy - Look Marvelous - Live Longer

But first it is important that you understand some of the fundamentals about aging and anti-aging.

Chapter 1
The Causes of Aging

"All would live long, but none would be old."
Benjamin Franklin

To live young forever has been man's quest throughout history. From among the first writings preserved in the clay tablets of Babylon we read of King Gilgamesh who searched for the secret of eternal life. The tablets tell us that he found it, but lost it to the snake – and died. Ponce de Leon searched for the fountain of youth – and never found it.

We are now beginning to understand aging.

Almost all life on earth blossoms with youth until it has reproduced and passed its genes on to the next generation. After that the flowers wilt and die, all animals age and die, and we humans begin to age and die. Yes, we begin to age while we are still in our 20's.

We age because the products of our metabolism, i.e., the "ashes" from the oxidation processes that produce energy in our cells accumulate faster than our aging endocrine system can remove them. This is because most of the cleansing hormones that surged through our youthful bodies begin to decrease as we begin to age. Some of these more critical hormones have decreased by about 10 to 30 percent as we enter our 30's.

The decreases become ever more dramatic as we enter successive decades of life. Most of our hormones have decreased by over 50% and some have been reduced to near zero as we enter our 70's. So we age.

Our muscles and bones weaken; our reaction time slows; we lose our agility: all combine to make us more susceptible to accidents. Our immune system weakens and makes us more susceptible to disease. And we die.

There are a dozen or so mechanisms of aging that have been theorized over time. The author believes that there are seven basic causes that combine to make us age:

1. Free radicals and other ashes of our metabolism, and environmental toxins build up in our cells and cause the cells to die without being able to reproduce themselves as they would normally do when you are younger.

2. Our endocrine system ceases to secrete sufficient quantities of certain enzymes and hormones to keep up with the cell's battles with the build-up of contaminants.

3. Our cells lose their ability to divide and replace themselves because they use up their allotted number of divisions (reach their Hayflick Limits as explained later).

4. Stress causes secretion of excessive cortisol which does significant damage.

5. Some of us have inherited flawed genes that cause or allow malfunctions.

6. Deficiencies in our diet limit the materials necessary for the cells to cleanse and repair themselves. Excesses in our diets adversely affect certain chemical reactions.

7. Lack of exercise causes atrophy of critical muscles that result in chemical imbalances and loss of strength and agility, which makes us prone to accidents.

All animals studied to date share these same causes of aging that they and we have inherited from our common evolution. Let's look at a little more detail for each of these 7 causes of aging.

1. Free Radicals, Lipofuscins, and Toxins

Mitochondria, located in almost all of your cells, convert the food you eat into energy. These products of your metabolism, i.e. this conversion to energy, also include "ashes" from the oxidation process that produces energy in our cells.

Some of these ashes are lipofuscins and free radicals that accumulate in our cells. These free radical molecules cause dangerous inflammation in the cell. Lipofuscins are the brown age spots we see on our skin. Similar "spots" and contaminants accumulate in our heart muscles, brains and elsewhere.

Most of the free radicals are a form of oxygen that "wants" to keep on "burning" with something. They attack various parts of the cell that they are in, including the cell walls and even the DNA. This eventually will cause the cell to become inoperative and die.

This oxidation is analogous to rusting. It results in a "rusting" of your arteries, which is partly responsible for the aging of your cardiovascular system.

Furthermore, many various types of environmental toxins find their way into our cells and frequently behave as free radicals and/or accumulate to the point of clogging the cell and impeding its operation. Some of the toxins that we encounter are potentially very harmful and can cause cancer, asthma, and various allergies. This can significantly reduce your quality of life. Their effects tend to speed up the aging process.

Our bodies naturally combat these processes by providing anti-oxidants from the food we eat and supplements that we may take. Such anti-oxidants include the well-known vitamins C and E that we get by eating certain fruits and vegetables and by supplementation.

And there are many more free radical fighters in the form of many dozens of other anti-oxidants and nutrients. The best fighters are the enzymes and hormones described below.

But we lose our best fighters as we age, and the free radicals eventually win their battles. We age and die.

But we can do something about free radicals as described later.

2. Hormone and Enzyme Decline

Our hormones regulate and control most of the functions of our bodies. Testosterone and estrogen, the major sex hormones in men and women respectively, give us the urge and ability to reproduce and continue the survival of our species.

But once we're past our reproductive prime, our hormone levels drop. This results in a lack of sex drive, insomnia, impotence, weight gain, and countless other potential health problems that significantly decrease our quality of life.

So we see that our hormone system was designed primarily for reproduction for the survival of the species. Our bodies produce high quantities of certain hormones and enzymes during our youth. These give us our youthful vitality, strength, and endurance. They help in the battles against free radicals and they help provide nutrients for cell repair. They keep our cells cleansed of the ashes of metabolism and environmental toxins.

As long as our bodies produce sufficient quantities of these enzymes and hormones, we stay young. But we and all plants and animals were designed to stay healthy until we have reproduced and reared our young. Mother Nature has little interest in us after we have passed our genes on to the next generation.

As we age past our prime reproductive years we are no longer capable of producing sufficient quantities of the enzymes and hormones required to keep our cells "young and fit." With too little of these substances, our cells begin to lose their battles against the free radicals and other destructive elements.

The cells begin to age, and die. The organs of which they are a part become ineffective. We become frail and die.

But we can do something about hormonal decline, as described in a later Chapter.

3. Telomere Erosion

As our cells age and become clogged with the ashes of metabolism and environmental toxins, they must replace themselves as they begin to become inoperative and begin to die. This is where telomeres come into play.

Our chromosomes are in the center nucleus of our cells. At each end of each of the paired chromosomes there is a telomere. It is analogous to the grommets at the ends of shoelaces. The telomeres keep the chromosomes organized.

As the cells age and become clogged the cell divides to reproduce its self. In so doing, it loses some of the telomere length.

Dr. Hayflick determined that most normal cells, after the initial rapid growth of the embryo, can divide about 50 more times after birth before their telomeres are too short for further divisions.

As our cells age they divide to produce new cells to replace themselves. But the more times that they divide, the less effective the cells become at reproducing themselves. Eventually their telomeres become too short for the cells to reproduce.

Baring poor nutrition and a poor environment, the telomeres of most of our cells may allow replacement for up to the age approaching 120 years.

Some have noted that this age limit is not unlike the limit of life span quoted in the Bible. This limit is now termed "The Hayflick Limit" because Dr. Hayflick was the one who discovered the telomere function.

Treatments that address the so-called normal aging mechanisms, and the standard treatments that provide age reversal, do not affect the Hayflick limit. This is a separate aging mechanism. Dr. Hayflick, and others, believes that we cannot live past 120 years of age.

But this is not necessarily true. We can do something about telomere erosion as is described later.

4. Stress

A study in 2004 first identified the direct link between stress and aging. Intense, long-term emotional strain and stress can make you get sick and grow old much faster than normal.

Stress is a normal part of life. Almost everything that happens to us put stress on our body. You can experience stress from your environment, your actions or inactions, the actions or inaction of others, your body aches, and even just your thoughts.

The human body is designed to experience stress and to react to it. Stress has a positive side in that it keeps us alert and ready to avoid danger. Stress becomes negative when you face continuous challenges without relief or relaxation between challenges. As a result, stress-related tension builds.

Our adrenalin system was designed to handle <u>acute stress</u> which is experienced in response to an immediately perceived threat, such as a lion about to eat us. During an acute stress response, the autonomic nervous system is activated and the body experiences increased levels of cortisol, adrenalin and other hormones that produce an increased heart rate, quickened breathing rate, and higher blood pressure. Blood is shunted to the big muscles to prepare the body to fight or run away.

This is known as the fight-or-flight response.

But our lives have changed. Now we are more likely to be subjected to chronic stress, which our bodies were not designed to handle.

Many of us experience chronic stresses caused by our modern lifestyle. It can be caused by everything from high-pressured jobs to loneliness to busy traffic. Such chronic stress can keep the body in a state of perceived threat. When this happens, our fight-or-flight response, which was designed to help us fight a few life-threatening situations spaced out over a long period, can wear down our bodies and cause us to become ill, either physically or emotionally.

Chronic stress, sometimes termed "distress", causes negative kinds of stress reactions. It occurs when stress continues without any relief. Distress can lead to physical symptoms including headaches, upset stomach, elevated blood pressure, chest pain, and problems sleeping.

Research shows that stress can also cause or worsen some diseases.

Stress causes the release of the so-called "stress hormones", of which cortisol is the primary. Chronically elevated levels of cortisol speed up the shortening of the telomeres and causes the cells to become ineffective in carrying out their purposes. And as previously described, we know that shortened telomeres speeds the body's deterioration and causes aging.

Cells with shortened telomeres cannot divide to form new cells so they die without replacing themselves. The tissue to which the cells are a part then ages much more quickly and soon dies. And then we die.

So stress prematurely shortens our telomeres and speeds up aging.

This helps explain the association between psychological stress and increased risk of physical disease. Unrelenting emotional pressure and stress definitely accelerates the aging process.

But we can do something to relieve chronic stress as described later.

5. Defective Genes

Defective genes are one of the factors affecting how fast and how well we age.

The Human Genome, which is a complete copy of the entire set of human genes, was basically decoded in 2003. With this decoding we now know, at least for many genes, which ones cause or allow, the major diseases of man. We can do a DNA profile analysis and detect an individual's inherited flaws. Such flaws or defective genes will indicate the diseases and/or the abnormalities that an individual may be susceptible to because of his or her genetic inheritance.

We have developed treatments to replace defective genes with some success. The first treatment occurred in 1999 and many more treatments have occurred since. All of these have been experimental and conducted by researchers. It will be a while longer before the procedures will be available to the general public.

Potential treatments are described in a later Chapter.

6. Dietary Deficiencies

Most of us in today's society do not experience dietary deficiencies unless or until we get older. But how fast, and well, we age will be affected when and if we do experience such deficiencies.

Our diets consist of five nutritional groups:
1. Proteins
2. Carbohydrates
3. Fats
4. Vitamins and supplements

5. Minerals

There are about 50 nutritional items within these groups that are necessary for good health. Age, gender, and overall health dictate how much of each of these nutrients you need.

We need to insure that we get all of the nutrients that we need from each of the 5 groups to prevent any deficiencies. Relatively simple blood tests can determine any deficiencies and can monitor for any developing deficiencies.

When deficiencies exist they can be treated by diet changes and with supplements as described in a later Chapter.

Chapter 2
Measurements of Aging

"Beauty is in the eye of the beholder and it may be necessary from time to time to give a stupid or misinformed beholder a black eye."
Miss Piggy

So we know what causes aging. But how do we measure age? How do we know if we are aging as slow as possible?

The most obvious measurement of age is our appearance. We can look at each other and usually give a pretty good guess of age. Gray hair, wrinkles, loose and thin skin, and extra weight are all apparent by just looking at an older person.

The easiest thing to see is weight and fat. The typical female at age 30 is 35% fat; at 80, 53%. Men are much more variable. But, as we age, almost all of us get increased fat and decreased muscle mass.

Our skin gets thinner, rougher, and less flexible. Our bones also get thinner and less dense: more fragile. Our major organs shrink and their functions decrease.

We all become slower and feebler. Our hair gets thinner, and gray. Yes, the effects of aging are visible. But, a more precise measurement of "biological" age can be obtained by measuring the levels of our various hormones.

Testing for the levels of several different hormones in the blood can help approximate your biological age and therefore give an indication of how well you are aging. Each of the blood elements that generally change with age can be inputted into a formula to calculate your biological age based on each of the hormones selected. Another formula called the Parameter Weighted Analysis (PWA) is then used to calculate the best representative biological age from the various element inputs.

The graft below shows how three of the hormones change with age for a male. Similar grafts can do the same for a female.

The most precise hormone measurement for age is DHEA. Blood levels of DHEA vary from person to person and average between 300 and 500 micrograms per deciliter of blood for twenty-year-olds.

DHEA and most all of the hormones decrease with age as depicted.

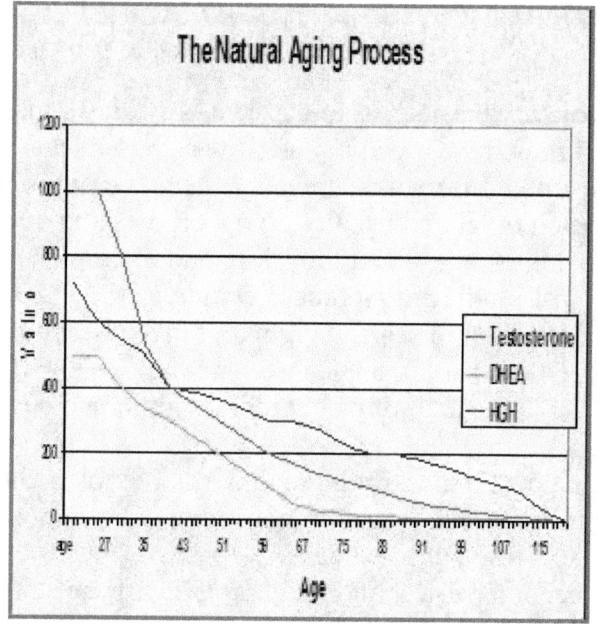

The fact that some people lose less DHEA than others can explain why some people age more slowly than others.

By measuring DHEA, and each of the other hormones in a blood test, we can calculate one's biological age as indicated by each of the hormones.

This is accomplished by comparing your current value for each of your key hormones with the typical values of the average person. It is noted, however, that adjustments must be made for individual differences.

This following chart shows the results using DHEA as the test element for a 51 year old man. His initial DHEA test indicated a biological age of about 5 years younger than his chronological age, suggesting that he was aging well.

However he wanted to age even slower and so he took treatment. After two months his biological age, according to this one element, i.e. his DHEA went down to under age 27.

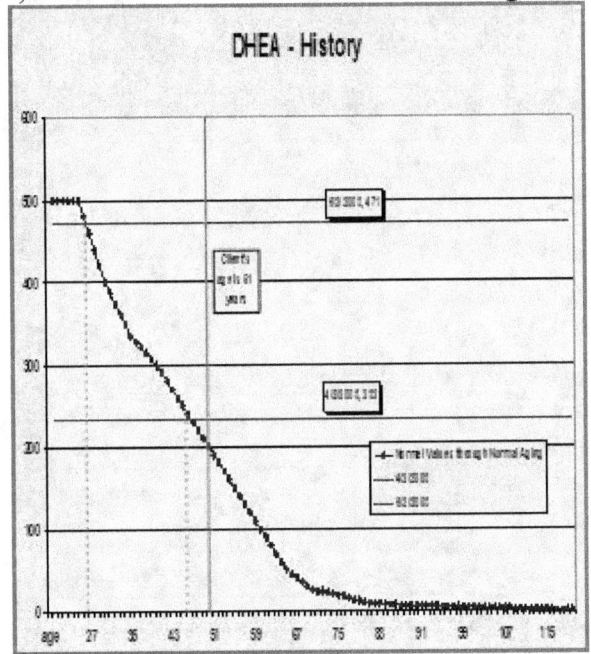

You can effectively reverse your biological age by up to 20 years by replacing your hormones to the levels you had in your more youthful days.

With such a program you can see significant results in about 6 months.

Another example is shown in the chart below for a 70 year old man who initially had a testosterone level of 120, which suggested a biological age of about 74. He was aging faster than normal.

After treatment, his testosterone level went up to 428 which indicated a biological age of less than 40.

He was aging poorly but treatment resulted in a very significant improvement in his biological age relative to this one element of his blood, i.e. testosterone.

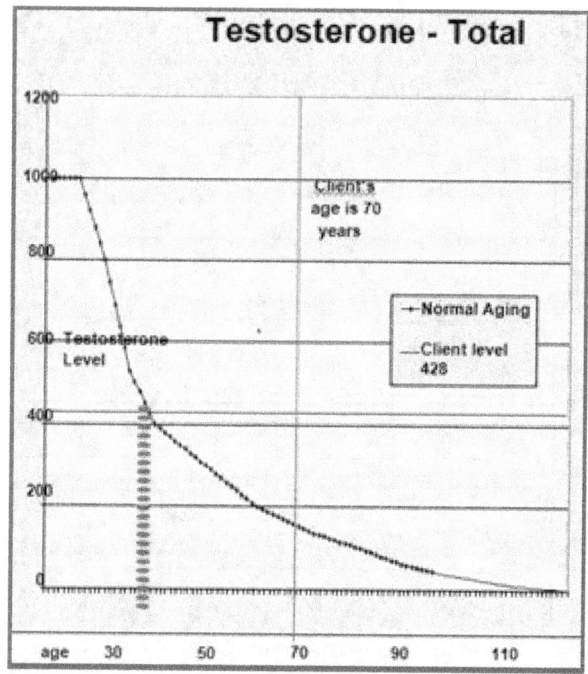

Biological age can indeed be assessed and treatments can slow down the aging process and provide a longer, higher quality lifespan.

The program for this procedure is termed Hormone Replacement Therapy (HRT) and is described in a later Chapter.

Chapter 3
Understanding Our Evolution

"I believe that our Heavenly Father invented man because he was disappointed in the monkey."
Mark Twain

Understanding our own human evolution provides insights into some details of our internal workings that enable us to do something about the disease of aging.

People reach their physical prime in their 20's and begin to age in their 30's. Some do both either a little earlier or a little later than others. We age at different rates because of our evolutionary heritage, our diets and our environment. Regardless of our religious beliefs, we must accept and understand our evolutionary heritage, and our relationship to other animals, in order to benefit from anti-aging procedures. We have to use our kinship to other animals and plants to manufacture the enzymes, hormones, and nutracuetials we need for anti-aging treatments.

All of us were created via evolution. This evolution was, depending on your beliefs and definition of God or Mother Nature, either random or by design of God. Either way, our evolution began from a single cell organism. We know this to be true from two sets of evidence.

Shared DNA

First, we share the same DNA as all the other plants and animals that evolved before us and along with us. We can all read each other's DNA. As proof of this, the human gene that instructs for the manufacture of human insulin has been spliced into bacteria. These bacteria produce 97% of the insulin, a human hormone, which is used today by diabetics.

The human gene that codes for human growth hormone (HGH) has also been spliced into bacteria. These bacteria produce the HGH used in the anti-aging programs.

Similar gene splicing is now used to produce food crops: over 15% of all corn, over 30% of all soybeans, and over 50% of all cotton produced during the last few years has been from genetically spliced DNA.

A genetically engineered salmon has been in development in fish farms for several years.

Using our understanding of the kinship among plants and animals, genes from a pig have been spliced into a tomato to retard spoilage of the tomato and thereby give it a longer "shelf life" between harvesting and retail sale in grocery stores.

Evolution in the Womb

The second set of evidence indicating that we evolved is the process we go through during our embryonic development in our mother's womb. All vertebrates show remarkable similarities as depicted in the drawings.

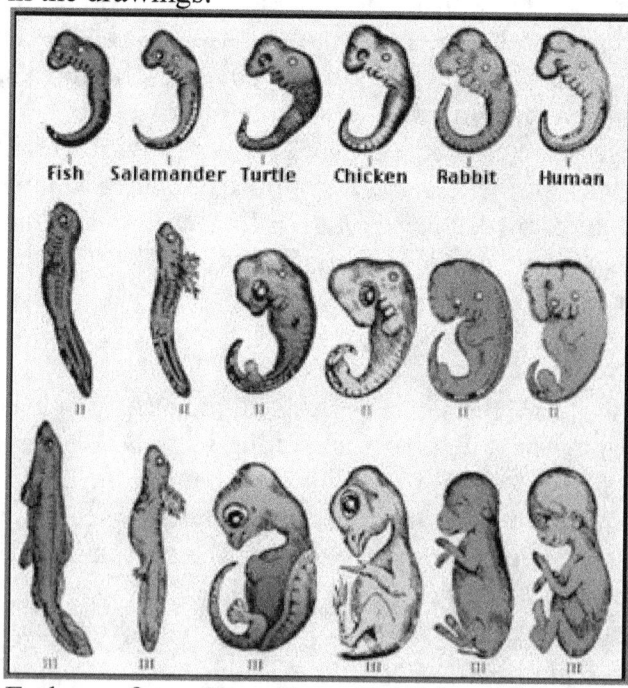

Embryos from Open Court Publishing Company

From these drawings you can see grooves looking like early gills in the early stage of development. These external views are matched on the inside by a series of paired gill pouches.

In fish the pouches and grooves eventually meet and form the gill slits, which allow water to pass from the pharynx over the gills and out of the body.

In the other vertebrates you see that the grooves and pouches disappear. In humans these early gill-like developments become the auditory canal of the outer ear and the Eustachian tube that goes from the middle ear to the nasal system.

The idea that embryonic development repeats the genealogy of the species is called recapitulation. This, however, is a distortion of the truth. But we do pass through some, though not all, of the embryonic stages that our ancestors passed through. Our genes do, however, instruct our embryonic development to follow a path from a one cell animal formed by the union of our father's sperm with our mother's egg. We as embryos then follow similar paths of other animals through the various stages of development.

As the embryo continues to grow, we can see early fish-like gills. Then we see a tail as one similar to the early amphibians, another stage in our evolution. We, as all mammals, go through the stage where all the mammal embryos look somewhat like a stage of our common mammalian ancestor.

Finally, we emerge from the womb as a human baby. But even then, and even now, we carry "old instructions" in our DNA that are no longer useful.

The fact that we still grow our useless appendix is a notable example.

The Human Genome Program

Perhaps the most important of all the recent projects that advance our understanding of aging was the decoding of the Human Genome in 2003. This project decoded the 20,000 or so genes that make up our human DNA. The instructions for "making" a human are presented in these genes.

The Genomes have also been decoded for other animals. It is totally clear that we do indeed share vary large percentages of the same DNA with the other animals of planet earth. And, surprisingly for some people, we share most of our DNA with some of the plants.

It is this recognition that we are evolved beings; and that we evolved with the animals and plants; and that we all share mostly the same DNA; that we can all read each others DNA; we can splice the DNA from plants and animals into other plants and animals, and into ourselves; and that provides us a capability to extend the youthful period of our lives today and promises to provide us immortal life in the foreseeable future.

We now know that aging is a treatable disease. It is not yet a curable disease, but it is indeed a treatable disease.

By treating our disease of aging today we may be able to extend our lives long enough to be able to take advantage of the cure that may be on the horizon.

Many researchers believe that the first immortals may be alive today.

Chapter 4
Anti-Aging Treatments
"Everything should be made as simple as possible, but not simpler."
Albert Einstein

You have choices of what you can do to slow your aging and increase longevity. Your choices range from the group of safe and well-used anti-aging programs to the riskier hormone replacement programs to more advanced unproven but promising programs, to a personalized program that may consist of personally tailored and selected elements from all of the choices.

Whichever program you choose, you should get started immediately to better insure that you will be around when the even more advanced programs currently in development become available. Many of the researchers believe that these programs have the potential for eternal life. That's something you shouldn't miss by just waiting around.

You can start your anti-aging longevity program by choosing from the following:

1. Understand and put into practice a proven basic anti-aging program specifically tailored to you. The future of medicine is in personal tailoring. These programs have 3 basic elements:

    a. Diet

    b. Supplements

    c. Exercise

This program is more effective and safer when you monitor your progress, and most importantly your safety, with periodic blood testing.

2. Understand and Practice Stress Therapy. It is not widely known how dramatically stress affects our health and aging.

3. Understand and consider personally tailored Hormone Replacement Therapy (HRT), which has proven very effective, but that may be risky.

4. Understand and consider personally tailored Hormone Precursor Therapy (HPT) which has proven effective but less so than HRT. It is, however considered much less risky than HRT, but a few still believe it may be somewhat risky since it has not had a long history.

5. Understand and consider the Calorie Restriction Program which can be effective but is far too uncomfortable for almost all people wishing to lead a normal life.

6. Understand and consider, if it applies to you, Gene Replacement Therapy.

7. Understand and participate in one or more of the as yet unproven "beta" programs resulting from the newly evolving technologies.

8. Develop your own Personally Tailored Program which can include your selections of various elements from all of the above.

Chapter 5
Proven Anti-Aging Program
"Be not the first by whom the new are tried, nor yet the last to lay the old aside."
Alexander Pope
1688-1744

Basic anti-aging programs have been developed and have evolved for ages. They have evolved as we learn more and more from various studies and experiments. These basic programs have been used long enough to prove their effectiveness and, most importantly, their safety.

They are not nearly as effective as the more advanced programs we discuss in subsequent Chapters; but they are safer than the newer, less tried programs.

These proven basic programs have 3 core elements: Diet, Supplements and Exercise. And if you are really serious, you should have you blood tested periodically to make sure that improvements are occurring and that no problems are developing.

Diet and Supplements

The aging process is slower for those who eat food with higher quantities of anti-oxidants and the nutrients needed for the body to continuously repair itself. A diet deficient in the necessary anti-oxidants and nutrients will age you faster.

You need to eat the right foods to prevent any deficiencies. You need to take supplements to insure that you get enough of the ingredients to enable you to age as slowly as possible.

In June 2009 the *American Journal of Clinical Nutrition* reported that multi-vitamins help women live 9.8 years longer.

Multi-vitamins can decrease the age-related DNA telomere shortening discussed above. Maintaining longer DNA telomeres with the use of multi-vitamins can significantly increase your healthy life span and likewise your longevity.

Poor nutrition together with too little physical inactivity was the second leading cause of death in 2000. Use of tobacco was the first.

Getting the correct nutrition becomes more difficult as we age. This is because we tend to eat less and therefore our vitamin and nutrient intake decreases.

Our ability to absorb vitamins and nutrients also decreases as we age. Taking the increased number and levels of medicines needed as we get older also interferes with the body's natural functions and leads to less efficiency in absorbing nutrients.

Furthermore, aging results in a loss of the ability to properly digest the nutrients from food so that they can be properly absorbed. This loss in absorption capability is mostly caused by the older body's inability to produce the enzymes needed for proper digestion and absorption.

The resulting lack of the proper vitamins and nutrients can lead to problems such as abdominal pain, bloating, diarrhea, flatulence (gas), skin ailments, arthritis, deteriorating eyesight, decreased bone mass, and hearing and memory loss; which all together causes us to age faster.

Nutrient deficiencies can also lead to more serious life-threatening problems such as calcification of the arteries and kidneys, various cancers, cardiovascular disease, high blood pressure, a degraded immune system, stroke, Alzheimer's, and a vastly increased rate of aging.

So the first thing that you need to do to increase your healthy longevity is to make sure that you eat a proper healthy diet and take the supplements needed for a long healthy life.

Many diet and supplement programs are currently available on the Internet.

Exercise

Along with your diet and supplement program, you know that you need to exercise to have better health and longevity. This is so obvious and well known that we will not repeat the same old urgings here. Just do it!

Get Started

You can select the proper diet and supplement program for you from the hundreds advertised online.

But don't wait; get started now!

Live Healthy - Look Marvelous - Live Longer

Chapter 6
Stress Relief Therapy
"In most cases stress is the root cause of death; illnesses are just the wrap up."
Yordan Yordanov

Stress is one of the worst culprits for speeding up the aging process.

Our bodies were just not designed to handle chronic stress that occurs when you face continuous problems without relief or relaxation between challenges.

Stress can become even more harmful when people use alcohol, tobacco, or drugs to try and relieve their stress. Unfortunately, instead of relieving the stress and returning the body to a relaxed state, these substances tend to keep the body in a stressed state and cause more problems.

Consider the following:

Stress causes forty-three percent of all adults to suffer adverse health effects.

Seventy-five percent to 90% of all doctor visits are for stress-related ailments.

Stress can cause headaches, high blood pressure, heart problems, diabetes, skin conditions, asthma, arthritis, depression, and anxiety.

The Occupational Safety and Health Administration (OSHA) declared stress a hazard of the workplace. Stress costs American industry more than $300 billion annually.

Emotional disorders are caused more than 50% of the time by chronic, untreated stress reactions.

Our adrenalin system was designed to handle <u>acute stress</u> which is experienced in response to an immediately perceived threat, such as a lion about to eat us. During an acute stress response, the autonomic nervous system is activated and the body experiences increased levels of cortisol, adrenalin and other hormones that produce an increased heart rate, quickened breathing rate, and higher blood pressure. Blood is shunted from the extremities to the big muscles, preparing the body to fight or run away.

This is known as the fight-or-flight response.

But our lives have changed. Now we are more likely to be subjected to chronic stress, which our bodies were not designed to handle.

Chronic stress occurs when the body experiences so many stressors that the autonomic nervous system rarely has a chance to activate the relaxation response, i.e. return to normal.

Chronic stress is often caused by our modern lifestyle. It is caused by everything from high-pressured jobs to loneliness to busy traffic. Such chronic stress can keep the body in a state of perceived threat. When this happens, our fight-or-flight response, which was designed to help us fight a few life-threatening situations spaced out over a long period, can wear down our bodies and cause us to become ill, either physically or emotionally.

In fact, it's estimated that up to 90% of doctor's visits are for conditions in which stress at least plays a role!

That's why it's so important to learn stress management techniques and make healthy lifestyle changes to safeguard from the negative impact of chronic stress.

The culprits that result from too much chronic stress are Cortisol and Adrenalin. They are both vital hormones that are secreted by the adrenal glands. Cortisol is the most damaging. It is involved in several important functions including:

1. Proper glucose metabolism
2. Regulation of blood pressure
3. Insulin release for blood sugar maintenance
4. Immune function
5. Inflammatory response

Although stress isn't the only reason that cortisol is secreted into the bloodstream, it has been termed "the stress hormone" because it's also secreted in higher levels during the body's so called fight or flight response to stress, and is responsible for several stress-related changes in the body.

Small and normal increases of cortisol have some positive effects:

1. A quick burst of energy for survival reasons
2. Heightened memory functions
3. A burst of increased immunity
4. Lower sensitivity to pain
5. Helps maintain better homeostasis in the body

So cortisol is an important and helpful part of the body's response to stress but it is important that the body quickly returns to normal following a stressful event.

When the body is no longer in perceived danger it normally returns to normal.

However, in times of chronic stress, when the body is in a constant state of physiological arousal over perceived threats that are numerous and not life-threatening, the body does not return to the normal state.

Higher and more prolonged levels of cortisol in the bloodstream caused by chronic stress have negative effects, including:

1. Impaired cognitive performance
2. Suppressed thyroid function
3. Blood sugar imbalances such as hypoglycemia
4. Decreased bone density
5. Decrease in muscle tissue
6. Higher blood pressure
7. Lowered immunity and inflammatory responses in the body, slowed wound healing, and other health consequences

Increased abdominal fat, which is associated with a greater amount of health problems than fat deposited in other areas of the body. Some of the health problems associated with increased stomach fat are heart attacks, strokes, and the development of metabolic syndrome, higher levels of "bad" cholesterol (LDL) and lower levels of "good" cholesterol (HDL), which can lead to other health problems!

To keep cortisol levels healthy and under control, the body's relaxation response should be activated after the fight or flight response occurs. You can learn to relax your body with various stress management techniques, and you can make lifestyle changes in order to keep your body from reacting to stress in the first place.

Stress Treatments

The following have been found by many to be very helpful in relaxing the body and mind and thereby aiding the body in maintaining healthy cortisol levels:

1. Breathing Exercises
2. Listening to Music
3. Exercise
4. Gardening, etc.
5. Sex
6. Self-Hypnosis
7. Yoga
8. Meditation

How to do each of these is rather obvious but you can learn more about each on the Internet.

I will describe in this brief eBook only what most experts think is the best: meditation.

Meditation

Many experts are convinced that stress greatly increases the rate at which we age. Most experts agree that stress of all kinds, mental, emotional, and physical, causes us to age.

Research and experience has shown conclusively that meditation is a potent stress reliever and therefore a potent anti-aging practice that can take years off your physiological and biological age.

Expert Eva Selhub, MD, Medical Director of the Mind/Body Medical Institute says, " *If we can affect the stress response, we can affect the aging process."* She says *"There's a reason why experienced meditators live so long and look so young."*

Dr. Robert Keith Wallace, one of the first scientists to study the effects of meditation on aging, found *that "subjects with an average chronological age of 50 years, who had been practicing Transcendental Meditation for over 5 years, had a biological age 12 years younger than their chronological age."*

That means a 55-year-old meditator had the physiology or biological age of a 43 year old.

Several of the subjects in the study were found to have a biological age 27 years younger than their chronological age. And this study has since been replicated several times.

History reveals many examples of seemingly "ageless" saints, dedicated to the practice of meditation, whose lives have demonstrated the enormous capacity of the human body to live much longer than today's normal average life span.

Other research also supports the value of meditation in keeping brains young. For example, we know that ordinarily the gray matter in our brains thins as we age. However, brain scans show that meditation actually helps preserve and add to the thickness of the gray matter, especially in areas of the brain associated with learning and motor skills.

Many scientists now believe that the brain can change and even grow; that it responds to use much as our muscles respond to exercise. There are many examples of people who have recovered functions lost during stroke or other adverse events.

This suggests that a meditator's brain may be healthier and more youthful than that of their non-meditating peers. Furthermore, the growth of gray cells in the motor skills part of the brain may have implications for balance and movement, also problem areas for elderly people.

That's why it's so important to learn stress management techniques and make healthy lifestyle changes to safeguard from the negative impact of chronic stress.

When are you going to start meditating?

The answer, of course, is when you want to increase your life span so you will be around when the new findings currently under development become available to extend your life even more.

Get started!

Chapter 7
Hormone Replacement Therapy

"Hormones, vitamins, stimulants and depressives are oils upon the creaky machinery of life. Principal item, however, is the machinery."
Martin H. Fischer

Hormone Replacement Therapy (HRT) is just what it says: You increase your decreasing hormone levels by injecting or otherwise ingesting hormones from outside your body.

The system is highly effective. I know for sure because I have tried it for the better part of a year.

The system however may be risky and therefore the US Government has taken steps to outlaw it. The Government's motivation to outlaw HRT was perhaps instigated initially to prevent human growth hormone, testosterone and other steroids from being used in sports - and especially to prevent being used by the young.

The first evidence that we can take actions that can **significantly** affect our aging process began to be realizable in 1989 when Dr. Daniel Rudman ran hormone replacement experiments on 12 men ages 61 to 81 and compared them to an age-matched control group. He turned their flabby, frail, fat-bulging bodies into their sleeker, stronger, younger selves. Rudman reported:

"The effects were equivalent in magnitude to the changes incurred during 10 to 20 years of aging."

In effect he had reversed their biological ages by 10 to 20 years. Dr. Rudman concluded:

"The overall deterioration of the body that comes with growing old is not inevitable."

Dr. Rudman published his historical findings in the prestigious *"The New England Journal of Medicine"* in June 1990.

Others have repeated and extended Rudman's tests and treatments.

It has been proven that Hormone Replacement Therapy (HRT) stops and reverses the "natural" aging process by replacing the body's hormones back to the levels experienced in youth.

Following Dr. Rudman's experiments, Dr. Edmund Chein has successfully completed age reversal treatments for hundreds of clients, a significant percentage of which are doctors.

Dr. Robert Goldman and Dr. Ronald Klatz formed the Institute of Anti-Aging in 1992 and now have over 20,000 members, many of which are doctors that are offering Anti-Aging treatments that incorporate hormone replacement therapy (HRT).

Other therapies using HRT had been practiced for many years:

1. Insulin hormone replacement for diabetes;

2. Estrogen hormone replacement for postmenstrual women (although recent tests were halted due to findings of adverse side effects);

3. Human growth hormone (HGH) replacement for growth stunted children.

The major hormones used in traditional HRT had been insulin for diabetes and estrogen with progesterone for postmenstrual women. The key hormones in the newer anti-aging programs have been human growth hormone (HGH) and testosterone.

Use of HGH has created a great deal of controversy, which is now at the point where a prescription is required for the hormone, and prescriptions are limited to those who have been shown by testing to be HGH deficient. The generally accepted level indicating deficiency is a blood serum of less than 350 ng/nl of insulin-like growth factor (IGF-1). IGF-1 is used for the measurement because it is a better indicator of the HGH levels than a direct measurement of HGH per se. HGH varies widely during the day while IGF-1, derived from HGH, remains more constant during the day.

Now it is well understood that our HGH levels decrease with age, and thus older people have HGH deficiencies relative to younger people. So all older people can be technically termed HGH deficient.

Several doctors have seized on this situation to offer HGH for age reversal purposes. The idea is that older people can again enjoy the benefits of the higher levels of HGH that they experienced in their youth. It is noted, however, that the body has feedback mechanisms that tend to balance the various hormones among each other, and that for HGH replacement therapy to be effective, and safe, additional hormones have to also be replaced to keep all of the key hormones in proper balance.

The more professional doctors that practice HRT provide such multiple hormones and do periodic blood monitoring to insure that all of the hormones stay in proper balance.

HGH and other hormone replacements can be dangerous if the proper procedures are not followed and properly monitored.

As Dr. Rudman and others have shown, HRT stops and reverses the natural aging process by replacing the body's hormones back to the levels experienced in youth. HRT can keep us biologically younger longer.

It is estimated that many thousands of people in the USA have experienced 10 years or more of effective biological age reversal. There are many more worldwide.

HRT has been proven to reverse biological age. But there are many who question its safety.

Test results have shown the following.

Benefits of Hormone Replacement Therapy	
Fitness	Percent Benefiting
Muscle Strength	88.0
Muscle Size	81.0
Higher Energy	86.8
Exercise Tolerance	81.0
Triceps Strength	60.7
Shoulder Strength	44.0
Buttocks	42.3
Back Flexibility	53.0
Muscle/Fat Ratio	25.0

Appearance	Percent Benefiting
Fat Loss	72.0
Skin Elasticity	73.0
Skin Texture	71.0
Skin Thickness	68.0
Sagging Checks	75.0
Wrinkled Face	71.0
Pouches Under Eyes	65.8
Skin Under Chin	62.5
Waist	40.0
Wrinkled Hands	41.6
New Hair Growth	38.0
Thicker Lips	25.0
Darkening Gray Hair	10.0

Other Benefits	Percent Benefiting
Emotional Stability	82.7
Immunity to Disease	73.0
Attitude	80.0
Healing Capacity	71.0
Sexual Potency	76.0
Duration of Penile Erection	62.0
Nighttime Urination	57.0
Hot Flashes	58.0
Memory	64.0
Lower LDL	*
Lower Triglycerides	*
Lower Blood Pressure	*
Osteoporosis	*
Arthritis Relief	*
Arterial Plaque	*
Heart Disease	*
Breast & Prostate Cancer	*

*Significant improvement, but not quantifiable due to differing interpretations of clients.

A proper HRT program can extend our youthful years and delay death; but there are risks.

These great results have been reported for many people, but not all. Some people experienced some benefits, but not all of the benefits. However, a detailed review of the hundreds of sets of test suggests that the therapy is effective and safe for many people, but can increase certain health risks for some people.

This has led to a great deal of controversy as to the safety of hormone replacement therapy (HRT). The US Government has declared it illegal for all but very limited situations.

The key ingredient to the benefits and potential adverse effects is Human Growth Hormone (HGH). The benefits can only be effectively obtained by injection; HGH is destroyed in the digestive system if taken orally.

HRT Ingredients

The ingredients for Hormone Replacement Therapy (HRT) must be prescribed by a certified medical professional. The ingredients from which a personalized therapy may be selected are described in a forthcoming eBook by the author. The book also describes the procedures for minimizing risk. You may contact him at info@PersonalHealthAnalysis.com

Bottom line: HRT is highly effective but may increase the likelihood of cancers and other health issues. It is currently offered by many practitioners that you can find on the Internet. But great caution is urged; it can be risky for some people.

Chapter 8
Hormone Precursor Therapy

"First, do no harm."
Thomas Sydenham
1624–1689

We will have to wait for further tests to see if the US Government will eventually allow the use of Hormone Replacement Therapy by making it legal for everyone.

Meanwhile you can get some of the benefits of HRT with hormone precursor therapy (HPT). This approach attempts to increase your decreasing hormones by making your own body increase its production.

Hormone Precursor Therapy (HPT) is considered primarily because it is an alternative to the more controversial Hormone Replacement Therapy (HRT).

HPT provides non-prescription supplements that stimulate the body to increase its own hormone production as opposed to HRT, whereby hormones are replaced by taking hormones from external sources.

It is perhaps much safer than HRT but it is no where near as effective as HRT.

It is however, probably the second most effective after HRT, of any other choices of the anti-aging longevity programs.

A potential problem with this approach is that the US Government is also considering outlawing some elements of this program.

But for now the benefits of HGH have proven to be so great for some people that the means of increasing one's HGH and other key hormones from within the body, without having to resort to illegal injections has been developed.

While HPT is neither as effective nor as fast in achieving results as the basic HRT programs, it does have several advantages:

It can be used for patients where tests indicate that the <u>HRT program may be too risky</u> for them.

It can be used for patients that are afraid of the HRT program.

It can be used after patients taking the HRT program have achieved the age reversal or heath position that they desire.

HPT is much less costly.

This program basically stimulates the body to increase its own hormone production levels. The program consists of providing the key precursors to each of the hormones and providing the nutracuetials and raw materials that the body needs to produce the higher levels of hormones.

A major purpose of HPT is to provide an alternative for those who strongly oppose the use of anabolic steroids or any illegal or banned substances. The HPT alternative is to help you achieve your goals without resorting to controversial or illegal or banned products.

The ingredients for Hormone Precursor Therapy (HPT) must be prescribed by a certified medical professional. The ingredients from which a personalized therapy is selected are described in a forthcoming book by the author. You may contact him at the publisher: <u>info@UnknownTruths.com</u>.

Chapter 9
Calorie Restriction Program

"We are creatures of our evolution. Recognize that; understand that; live that and you will live healthier and longer."
Walter Parks

Calorie Restriction (CR) has been proven very effective. Many believe that calorie restriction is the number one way we can extend longevity. The belief is based on tests with various animal studies and tests that have shown CR can probably extend your life expectancy by up to 50 percent.

But not everyone would want to live, must less live longer, on such a restricted regimen. Understand the facts and then decide if this is the way you want to live even if it can extend your life by 50 percent.

Calorie Restriction (CR) slows aging and extends life by taking advantage of a newly discovered chemical pathway we "inherited" from our ancient ancestors. Our bodies were designed not to waste calories in times of famine. CR makes the body get really efficient. It turns on the sirtuins pathway.

The sirtuins pathway evolved to recognize that we should not do our natural calling to make babies when food supplies are limited. It adjusts your metabolism to make you live longer, apparently waiting until food supplies are more available for you to work on the survival of your species.

During these times of restricted calories we experience fewer waste products in our cells, because our cells are processing less food and thus the cells live longer.

CR also helps organisms cope with periods of famine in other ways that we have inherited from our ancestors. Pankaj Kapahi, an assistant professor at the Buck Institute for Age Research, in Novato, California, says: "You can imagine that whenever food is limited in the wild, the animal goes into a sort of stasis. Then, when food is abundant, it will come out of that state and start eating so it can reproduce."

By shutting down growth and reproductive processes when food is scarce, the animal's body can focus all of its metabolic resources on survival by improving the efficiency of energy production and the clearance of the ashes of metabolism and damaged cellular proteins.

Kapahi discovered that inhibiting the Target of Rapamycin (TOR) signaling pathway extends the life span of a fruit fly. The TOR pathway is a protein that regulates cell growth, cell proliferation, cell motility, cell survival, protein synthesis, and transcription.

It controls cell growth in response to nutrient availability. The TOR integrates the input from upstream pathways, including insulin, growth factors and mitogens (a chemical that signals a cell to commence cell division).

By eating less, modern humans might engage these ancient pathways to extend life span.

Some have already begun.

The Evidence for CR Effectiveness

Scientists have known for decades that caloric restriction slows aging and extends life span in organisms ranging from yeast to mice.

In laboratory animals such as fruit flies, roundworms, and mice, caloric restriction switches biochemical pathways on or off, resulting in higher insulin sensitivity, decreased inflammation, enhanced cardiovascular functioning, reduced muscle wasting with age, and improved resistance to cellular stress.

Not only is normal aging slowed, but calorie-restricted animals are also less likely to develop age-associated diseases such as diabetes and cancer.

It has been found that life spans of yeast, worms and flies are increased 2 to 3 fold with calorie restriction.

In mice fed a calorie-restricted diet, these effects translate to a greater than 30% increase in life span.

Studies in primates and humans have been slower to obtain results because their longer life span takes much more time.

There are however dangers with CR. You may not get the proper amounts of critical nutrients. The lack of needed nutrients can create more damage than the good that CR provides. Therefore you must be careful to insure that the foods that you do eat contain the needed nutrients.

People that have started CR not only slowed their aging, but actually reversed their biological age.

Research indicates that a 30 percent decrease in daily caloric intake is sufficient to get effectiveness.

With CR it is possible to extend your life by 20 years or more!

Tests with mice have shown that Calorie Restriction slows down the onset of cell senescence. Cell senescence is the point at which a cell can no longer replicate itself. All cells eventually die and when cells cannot replace themselves the tissue of which they are a part will die and then you die.

Calorie Restriction accomplishes this because it helps protect the telomeres. And we know from the previous discussions that if we can prevent telomere erosion, that we can live longer.

Following a calorie-restricted diet has also been shown to slow the effects of aging on the muscles, brain and heart. New findings show that cutting calories may also reduce chronic disease by slowing age-related changes in the genes of the heart.

It was also found that the effects of Calorie Restriction seem to be significant even if Calorie Restriction is started later in life and maintained for only a relatively short period of time.

We are learning more and more about CR. It appears that CR changes the way in which your cells remove damaged components and recycle the materials into new replacement parts.

We know from the previous discussions that the ashes of metabolism build up in our cells and degrade their functions and eventually cause them to die. The changes in removal of these ashes enabled by CR helps the cells live longer.

Calorie restriction also provides many other benefits by greatly lowering the risk for most degenerative conditions of aging.

In addition, studies in invertebrates have provided compelling evidence for the vital role of TOR signaling in caloric restriction and aging. Richard A. Miller, a professor at the University of Michigan, and coworkers reported that TOR extends the life span of mice. These findings "make TOR the first protein that has been shown to modulate life span in each of the four organisms most commonly used to study aging: yeast, worms, flies, and mice."

Researchers think that when TOR signaling is blocked, whether from genetic mutation, Rapamycin treatment, or caloric restriction, cells slow growth by decreasing protein synthesis, ribosome production, and amino acid transport. Simultaneously, the organism becomes more resistant to some forms of stress. The recycling of damaged cellular components increases.

Although the TOR pathway has captured much of the limelight in recent years, other biochemical pathways such as the insulin/insulin-like growth factor 1, AMP kinase, and Sir2 pathways likely play supporting parts, at least under some conditions.

Researcher Kaeberlein says: "The conclusion that people are coming to is that all of these signaling pathways that respond to growth factors and nutrients are talking to each other. I think a very appealing hypothesis is that TOR coordinates several of the responses that go along with caloric restriction, including turning down protein synthesis and modulating the response to glucose and the insulin pathway."

A research team led by Richard Weindruch, a professor at the University of Wisconsin, Madison, reported groundbreaking findings from a 20-year study of caloric restriction in a close human cousin, the rhesus monkey.

The monkeys, which were placed on calorie-restricted diets at 7 to 14 years old, are now in old age. The effects of caloric restriction were dramatic. Calorie-restricted monkeys not only appeared younger, but also showed significantly reduced incidences of diabetes, cancer, and cardiovascular disease, as well as age-associated brain atrophy and muscle wasting. Compared with calorie-restricted monkeys, control animals had a threefold higher rate of death from an age-related cause.

At the time of the report, the calorie-restricted monkeys had an 80% survival rate, whereas only 50% of the control animals were still alive. Although Weindruch and coworkers won't know for another 15 years whether caloric restriction extends the maximum life span of rhesus monkeys (normally about 40 years), these results clearly demonstrate that caloric restriction lengthens the average life span of a primate species.

The findings are encouraging for the prospects of extending human longevity through caloric restriction.

Luigi Fontana, a research associate professor of medicine at Washington University in St. Louis and director of the Division of Nutrition & Aging at the Italian National Institute of Health in Rome, has been studying members of a group of people who voluntarily restrict calorie intake to improve health and slow aging.

Results are encouraging. "The data suggest that most of the metabolic adaptations to caloric restriction in mice and monkeys are also occurring in humans," Fontana says.

Further: "On the basis of their metabolic profiles, [the group] have practically zero risk of developing cardiovascular disease or stroke. We've also measured the elasticity and efficiency of the left ventricle and found that these people have hearts that are 15 years younger in terms of biology," he says.

In addition, "preliminary data suggest that many hormones and growth factors implicated in cancer are also reduced," he says.

Even knowing that caloric restriction improves human health and could extend life span, most people probably won't be rushing to adopt CR.

It's just too restrictive.

But even if most people do not want to subject themselves to such a restrictive regimen, the work could help scientists to better understand, and ultimately prevent a range of age-related diseases in humans and increase our lifespan.

A human study by John O. Holloszy, a professor of medicine at Washington University in St. Louis, published earlier this year noted that 18 people who had been practicing CR for three to 15 years showed dramatically reduced risk of developing diabetes or clogged arteries.

Well that's an introduction to Calorie Restriction. Is it for you?

Chapter 10
Gene Replacement Program

"We've got ninety-nine per cent the same genes as any other person. We've got ninety per cent the same as a chimpanzee. We've got thirty percent the same as a lettuce. Does that cheer you up at all? I love about the lettuce. It makes me feel I belong."
Caryl Churchill

Gene therapy is just now becoming exciting news. It will soon become the key to medicine. Its potential is limitless now that we have decoded the human genome.

We have entered the era where man can change his genes even in mature life. The promise is that some diseases normally associated with aging will be curable and reversible. Some already have been, and more and more are being demonstrated, as we better understand the Human Genome and gene vectoring techniques.

Researchers have used several different approaches for correcting faulty genes.

Understanding Genes

You can perhaps better understand defective genes by understanding a few terms. DNA (deoxyribonucleic acid) is the body's material that contains your genetic information and is present in each of the body's cells. DNA is made up of four similar chemicals that are called bases. The four bases are abbreviated A, T, C, and G. Sequences of these bases are repeated over and over in pairs.

Particular sequences of these bases make up a gene. Each gene provides coded instructions for making everything the body needs, especially proteins. We humans have about 25,000 genes.

The genes are packaged on very long strands of double helixes that are tightly wrapped to form chromosomes. Humans have 23 pairs of chromosomes for a total of 46. One pair make up the sex

53

chromosomes that determine whether you are male or female and provide instructions for additional body characteristics associated with your sex. The remaining 22 pairs are autosomal chromosomes that determine the rest of the body's makeup.

Each chromosome makes up one very large DNA molecule.

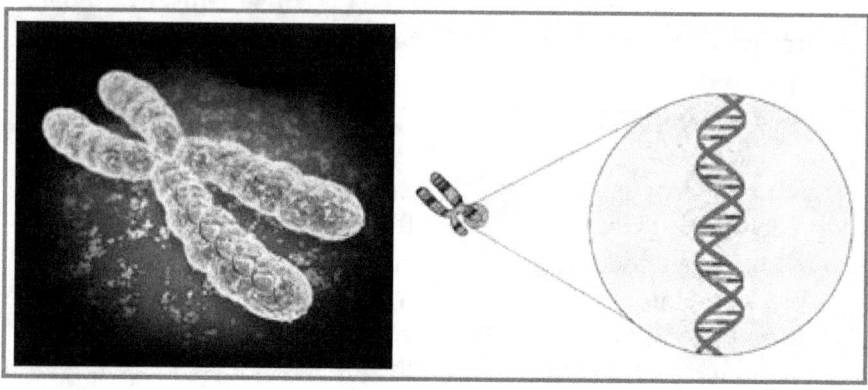

A gene is a segment of DNA that is coded to build a protein. Proteins are chains of chemical building blocks called amino acids. Various proteins are composed of anywhere from just a few amino acids in its chain or it could have several thousands.

Proteins enable most of what the body does including digestion, making energy, growing and keeping us immune from diseases.

The human genome has not yet been completely decoded so the functions of many of the genes are still unknown. However, with certain genes that we do know about, we have been able to replace defective genes with "good" genes by several different researchers.

And genetic materials, not complete genes per se, have also been successfully used to achieve "genetic cures" in many additional cases.

A defective gene occurs when the particular order of the pairs of A, T, C, and G gets switched, dropped, or repeated. This changes the coding for one or more genes creating a genetic mutation. The mutation may cause a disease or it may be harmless.

Mutations may occur in other ways such as if parts of a chromosome breaks off, switches with part of another chromosome, or becomes swapped within the same chromosome. If any of these or other mistakes occurs then mutations occur in the gene coding.

And sometimes the chromosome pair may lose one side or have a third chromosome instead of the normal pair.

The chromosomes and genes are more susceptible to errors when the telomeres grow short with age and can no longer keep the chromosomes organized, as previously discussed.

But we are learning how to "fix" some of these "mistakes" or mutations.

Gene Repair Techniques

The most common approach is to insert a normal gene within the genome to replace a nonfunctional gene.

Another technique is termed homologous recombination, where an abnormal gene could be swapped for a normal gene.

The abnormal gene may also be repaired through selective reverse mutation, which returns the gene to its normal function.

The researcher may alter the regulation, i.e. the degree to which a gene is turned on or off, of a particular gene.

The basic way such gene alterations are achieved is that a normal gene is inserted into the genome to replace an abnormal, disease-causing gene.

The insertion is with a carrier molecule called a vector. The vector used for the most part is a virus that has been genetically altered to carry normal human DNA.

Viruses have evolved a way of delivering their genes into human cells for their reproduction. They do not have complete reproduction systems within themselves.

Researchers take advantage of this capability of the viruses to deliver the gene that they want to insert.

The technique is to modify the virus by replacing parts of its internal materials with the gene you want it to insert. The virus is then inserted into the appropriate human location to "infect" the human with this altered virus. The virus then does what it normally does: it unloads its genetic material containing the therapeutic human gene into the target cell.

The generation of a functional protein product from the therapeutic gene restores the target cell to a normal state.

Various types of viruses have been used as such vectors.

Adenoviruses have been used. These are a class of viruses with double-stranded DNA genomes that cause respiratory, intestinal, and eye infections in humans. The virus that causes the common cold is an adenovirus.

Retroviruses have also been used. These are a class of viruses that can create double-stranded DNA copies of their RNA genomes. These copies of its genome can be integrated into the chromosomes of host cells. Human immunodeficiency virus (HIV) is a retrovirus.

Adeno-associated viruses have also been used. These are a class of small, single-stranded DNA viruses that can insert their genetic material at a specific site on chromosome 19.

Herpes simplex viruses have also been used. These are a class of double-stranded DNA viruses that infect the cell type of neurons. Herpes simplex virus type 1 is a common human pathogen that causes cold sores.

Nonviral options have also been used. The simplest method is the direct introduction of the desired DNA into target cells. This approach is limited in its application because it can be used only with certain tissues and requires large amounts of DNA.

Other nonviral techniques have also been used. A technique to pass the desired DNA through the target cell's membrane has been used. The technique of chemically linking the DNA to a molecule that will bind to special cell receptors has also been used.

Researchers also are experimenting with introducing an additional chromosome into the cell to be changed. This 47th chromosome would exist parallel to the 46th chromosome. It would be a large vector capable of carrying substantial amounts of genetic code, and scientists anticipate that, because of its construction and autonomy, the body's immune systems would not attack it. A problem with this potential method is the difficulty in delivering such a large molecule to the nucleus of a target cell.

Current Status of Gene Therapy

Treatments with gene therapy have been allowed but the Food and Drug Administration (FDA) has not yet approved any human gene therapy product for general public use. It is limited to research.

The first trial was in 1990. But gene therapy suffered a major setback with the death of Jesse Gelsinger in 1999. He was only 18 years old. He was participating in a gene therapy trial for Ornithine Transcarboxylase deficiency (OTCD). He died from multiple organ failures 4 days after starting the treatment. His death is believed to have been triggered by a severe immune response to the adenovirus carrier that was used.

Another major blow came in January 2003, when the FDA placed a temporary halt on all gene therapy trials using retroviral vectors because two additional deaths of patients being treated for the so-called "bubble baby syndrome".

The FDA eased the ban in April of 2003.

More Recent Developments in Gene Therapy

Nanotechnology was used in genes for the first time in 2009 to destroy cancer cells.

The technique is to wrap the desired genes in microscopic nano-particles. These "wraps" are then taken up by cancer cells, but not by their healthy neighbor cells. Once inside, the genes stimulated the production of a protein which destroys the cancer.

The researchers believe that the technology would be particularly relevant for people with cancers that are inoperable because they are close to vital organs and for cancers that have spread.

Although it has only been tested in mice so far, the researchers hope for human trials very soon.

What You Can Do Now

If you suspect that you have inherited any defective genes you can get a DNA analysis to check out any genes that you suspect may be defective or that may carry unwanted characteristics. Depending on the severity of the consequences of the defective gene or genes, you may be able to find a researcher that could include you in his program.

Remember you need to do whatever is necessary to insure that you survive to be available for the anti-aging treatments that are coming available over the next decade or so.

Chapter 11
Telomerase Treatment
"How old would you be if you didn't know how old you were?"
Satchel Paige

Daily life results in our cells becoming clogged with the ashes of metabolism and environmental toxins. To remedy this problem the cells divide and replace themselves before they become inoperative and begin to die. This works fine when we are young.

But each time they divide they loose a part of their telomeres at the ends of their chromosomes that keep them organized. When the telomeres become too short the cells have less ability to divide and so we age. Eventually the cell uses up its allotted number of divisions, called the Hayflick Limit, as previously explained.

Effects of Telomere Shortening

As the telomeres begin to get too short for our cells to be replaced, our skin gets thinner, rougher, and less flexible. Our bones also get thinner and less dense; more fragile. Our major organs shrink and their functions decrease.

Our physical measurements are also an indicator of our aging because of the telomere erosion. Our face and head usually get larger. Our neck grows extra folds and we add an extra chin or two. Our bodies begin to bend over and sometimes lose calcium in the bones and grow shorter. Our bodies lose their youthful taper. We lose our skin tone.

Our physical abilities decline. We cannot run as fast, if we can run at all. We cannot lift the heavy weights that we used to be able to do. We cannot endure physical work as long.

Our sexual performance approaches being just a memory as we grow older and older. Eventually even our memories fade.

We all become slower and feebler. Our hair gets thinner and gray.

Let's understand more about the telomere cause of aging. Dr. Hayflick has shown that we have a built-in death date of about 120 years, if diseases or accidents do not get us earlier. The point at which our cells have divided a fixed number of times until their telomeres become too eroded sets this death date. It has been termed the "Hayflick Limit."

Resetting the Death Clock

But tests over the past few years have indicated that the "Hayflick Limit" may be extended by the use of an enzyme that causes the "organizing genes" at the ends of the chromosomes (the telomeres) to re-grow. This enzyme is called telomerase.

A few years ago cancer researchers noted that some cancer cells divide and reproduce extremely fast, and many more times than the Hayflick Limit. It was learned that these cancer cells secrete an enzyme named <u>telomerase</u>. Telomerase causes the telomeres at the ends of the chromosomes to grow such that their cells can continue to divide.

These cancer cells appear immortal.

The researchers became both excited and concerned: excited that cells could become immortal; concerned that such cells would always become cancerous.

A series of experiments involving various cells, including human cells from the foreskin of circumcised infants, proved that telomerase could be used without inducing cancer. These human cells were injected with telomerase and grew longer telomeres. There was no cancer. The cells continued to divide many times beyond their Hayflick Limit. So far the cells have divided the quantity of times equivalent to a human life of over 1500 years.

These human cells appear immortal.

Telomerase therapy promises to extend life beyond the 120-year Hayflick Limit.

Genetically engineered and cloned rats have now reproduced for several generations. Some of them have had their life spans increased to that equivalent to 150 human years.

It is noted that our bodies produce telomerase while we are rapidly growing embryos in the womb. However, our bodies cease to produce telomerase after birth except possibly for sperm cells.

Some believe that we can find a way to turn the genes that produced telomerase when we were embryos back on.

Telomerase treatments on human cells in the laboratory have indicated that telomerase can make cells immortal. Doctors and researchers involved in these treatments are reporting that it is their belief that death is not inevitable.

Some areas of the body suffer more "stress" than do other parts, and therefore use up their Hayflick Limit sooner. An example is the rough skin on the hands and necks of field workers that have experienced long exposures to the sun. The skin cells continuously divide to build new cells to replace themselves; to correct the continuing damage, and thus use up their Hayflick limits. The consequence is that the back of the neck and the tops of the hands appear to age faster than does the rest of the (unexposed) skin.

Our first significant use of telomerase treatments will likely be to rejuvenate such sun-damaged skin. Other telomerase treatments will be offered after the treatments on sun-damaged skin prove their effectiveness, and safety.

We are still some years away from being able to use telomerase treatments for most of the more complex procedures. Extensive tests are required.

Some scientists believe that telomerase therapy will some day offer eternal life.

It is interesting to note that Time Magazine's cover of February 21, 2011 boldly states: "2045: The Year Man Becomes Immortal."

Stay tuned. Telomerase treatments may be closer than some believe.

Chapter 12
Anti-Aging Developments for the Future
"Life is a moderately good play with a badly written third act."
Truman Capote

We have long accepted the fact that we will die. But more and more researchers are beginning to believe that death is not inevitable. Maybe we can improve what Capote called the third act.

As new technologies and findings to increase longevity are developed, there is a growing need for test participants, that is guinea pigs.

Such opportunities are for those who are more interested in potential effectiveness than safety.

I guess I may consider such a program when I suspect that I do not have much life left. The problem is people at that late stage are usually not acceptable in the "beta" test programs.

I do tend to agree with those who believe that we could possibly become immortal.

There are many very advanced ongoing research projects that are beginning to show promise.

The CGK733 Synthesized Molecule

One such project is from a team of South Korean scientists. They report that they have created a newly synthesized molecule, named CGK733 that can make cells younger.

"All cells face an inevitable death as they age. On this path, cells became lethargic and in the end stopped dividing but we witnessed that CGK733 can block the process," Professor Kim Tae-kook reported.

He further stated: *"We also found the synthetic compound can reverse aging by revitalizing already lethargic cells. Theoretically, this can give youth to the elderly via rejuvenating cells."*

Kim expects that the CGK733-empowered drugs that keep cells youthful far beyond their normal life span will be commercialized in less than 10 years.

"We have the magnet associated technology to identify molecular targets inside living cells, which allowed us to examine the mechanisms of CGK733 directly," Kim said.

"Unlike other research teams that must make candidate materials for drugs without being able to see their intra-cell activities; we know the precise mechanism of CGK733. So we have the better chance of making a success of the substance," he continued.

The Wistar Project

Another activity aimed towards future longevity improvements is from researchers at The Wistar Institute. They have defined a key target of an evolutionarily conserved protein that regulates the process of aging. The study provides fundamental knowledge about key mechanisms of aging that could point toward new anti-aging strategies and cancer therapies.

Scientists had long known that a class of proteins called sirtuins promotes fitness and longevity in most organisms ranging from single-celled yeast to mammals. At the cellular level sirtuins protect genome integrity, enhance resistance to adverse stresses, and antagonize senescence. However, the underlying molecular mechanisms have remained poorly understood.

The Wistar team, led by senior author Shelley Berger, Ph.D., Hilary Koprowski Professor at The Wistar Institute, demonstrated for the first time a molecular target for a member of this class, Sir2, in regulation of aging in yeast cells.

Conclusions on Future Projects

These are just 2 of the many ongoing projects. It is easy to conclude that we will find an answer to immortality; perhaps even before 2045 as suggested by the ***Time Magazine*** cover of February 21, 2011.

We know that aging saps our strength and ability to enjoy life; it cripples us and eventually kills us. Tens of millions die from age-related conditions each and every year. Comparatively few people know that degenerative aging can be slowed with diet and lifestyle choices, medicines, nutracuetials and some of the programs outlined above.

The future of medicine is in personal tailoring. We are all different because of our genetics, our diets, and our past and current lifestyles. You can optimize your current and future health by defining and taking needed medications, vitamins, and other supplements and treatments tailored to your specific health profile.

You need to understand aging and what you can do about it.

You need to develop and practice your personal anti-aging longevity program.

Chapter 13
Your Anti-Aging Longevity Program

"The problem with doing nothing is not knowing when you're finished."
Benjamin Franklin

We are all different and we all have different opinions about anti-aging and longevity programs. Some people are doubtful about the long-term benefits of the anti-aging programs that have been discussed above. You should know, however, that many of us have already achieved biological age benefits equivalent to 10 to 20 years using these programs.

The approach you choose for your program will be your decision and that decision will be based on what you know and/or believe about aging and longevity. But whatever approach you choose, you can most likely benefit from the information presented in this book.

The future of medicine is in personal tailoring. We are all different because of our genetics, our diets, and our past and current lifestyles. You can optimize your current and future health by defining and taking needed medications, vitamins, and other supplements and treatments tailored to your specific health profile. Personally tailored diets and exercises, tailored to your specific health profile, will further improve your health and its effect on your quality and length of life.

America, and indeed the world, is aging. As the Baby Boomers retire over the next several years, they will significantly change society. Their diseases that come with aging will drastically affect the health care industry. But you can do something about it:

Aging Is A Treatable Disease.

You can begin to treat your diseases of aging and other disease and disability problems by determining your personal health profile and by making needed changes to your specific medical and lifestyle needs. Your current and future health can be improved by taking 3 steps:

1. Thoroughly understand your personal health profile. A group is currently developing a Personal Health Analysis system to help you.

2. Taking a specialized Blood Test at your local Quest Diagnostics office, LabCorp or some other blood test facility can provide additional details for your personal health profile.

3. Providing blood for a Personalized DNA Analysis. This is usually not necessary unless you have reason to believe that you may have genes that make you prone to certain diseases.

A proper assessment of one's health profile requires the measurement, analysis, and evaluation of an enormous number of parameters. It requires an understanding of the cause and effects of each of these parameters, and the interactions of each of these parameters with each other, and with the group of parameters. It requires a detailed understanding of the body's feedback mechanisms and their temporal stabilization frequencies.

Such an analysis is beyond the ability of any human; the massive data base capability and the massive computational capability of a properly designed and programmed computer are required to development one's health assessment.

DNA Profile Analysis
The analysis program can determine if part of the blood drawn for the blood tests should also be used for selected DNA analysis if abnormal genetic disorders are indicated.

Additional analysis can also be performed for any specific gene searches that you may request. This will be an optional feature that involves an additional computer questionnaire that is now in development. This program can reference a listing of all currently mapped genes from the Human Genome (HG) that may significantly affect your health profile.

Interactive screens are being developed to enable you to search for any disease or problem in which you may have a concern. Selective icons will allow you to continue your probing to any levels you choose.

You are likely to find it interesting to spend time "playing" with this very informative program when its development is complete.

Medical Exam

See your doctor or health care specialists to establish the basis for your health care activities.

Live Healthy - Look Marvelous - Live Longer

Epilog
The Search for Eternal Life
"The average man, who does not know what to do with his life, wants another one, which will last forever."
Anatole France
1844 – 1924

The first immortal human may be living today.

Some scientists believe this.

Are we on the verge of learning how to live young forever? Are we realizing one of mankind's most ancient quests? Are we finding what eluded King Gilgamesh of ancient Babylon? Are we about to find Ponce de Leon's Fountain of Youth?

In 1786, life expectancy was 24 years. Better diets and some medical innovations allowed it to double to 48 years in the next 100 years.

Modern medicine has now increased life expectancy to over 76 years.

Future medicine promises to increase it to over 100 <u>during your lifetime</u>.

"Over half the baby boomers here in America are going to see their hundredth birthday and beyond in excellent health," says Dr. Ronald Klatz of the American Academy of Anti-Aging. *"We're looking at life spans for the baby boomers and the generation after the baby boomers of 120 to 150 years of age."*

The causes of aging are finally being understood.

Comparatively few people are aware of the many serious scientific efforts, presently underway, aimed at understanding and intervening in the aging process in order to one day reverse its effects.

There are things that you can do today to help insure that you will live long enough to take advantage of the medical breakthrough now being developed.

You need to get started on your personal anti-aging longevity program now so you will be around to take of advantages of all of these developing programs.

Join the race to be among the first immortals!

About the Author

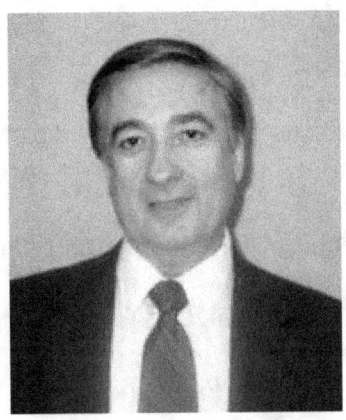

Hi! Thanks so much for your interest in my books!

My principal interests are true stories of the unusual or of the previously Unknown or unexplained. I have occasionally also written some fiction.

I was born in Memphis Tennessee and grew up in Saltillo Mississippi, a small town near Tupelo Mississippi. High School life was dominated by watching the rise of our local Elvis. I was editor of the High School Paper and had plenty to write about. I guess this was the beginning of my writing career.

After graduating from Mississippi State University as an aerospace engineer I moved to Orlando Florida and worked for Lockheed Martin for 24 years. I advanced from an aerospace engineer to a Vice President of the Company and President of the Tactical Weapons Systems Division.

Education Activities

I continued my education throughout my career with a MBA degree from Rollins College and with Post Graduate Studies in Astrophysics at UCLA; Laser Physics at the University of Michigan; Computer Science at the University of Miami; Gas Dynamics at MMC and Finance and Accounting at the Wharton School, University of Pennsylvania.

While at Mississippi State University I was on the President's Honor List and in the honor societies of Tau Beta Pi, Sigma Gamma Tau and Blue Key.

I received a scholarship from Delta Air Lines based on my academics and performance.

I was in ROTC and the Arnold Air Society where I participated and toured as a member of the precision Drill Team. I also attended the summer survival training at Hamilton Air Force Base in California.

I was selected for Who's Who among Students in American Universities and Colleges.

I was a speaker for several technical organizations including the American Institute of Aeronautics and Astronautics.

After retirement from Lockheed I formed Parks-Jaggers Aerospace Company and sold it 4 years later.

After selling my aerospace company I formed Quest Studios, Quest Entertainment and Rosebud Entertainment to make films at Universal Studios. I produced 10 films, directed 7 films and wrote 5 film scripts produced at Universal Studios.

I won the National Association of Theater Owners Show South Producer of Tomorrow Award.

I then formed UnknownTruths Publishing Company to publish true stories of the unusual or of the previously Unknown or unexplained. These include books about past events so unbelievable that most people have relegated them to "myths".

I have published 34 books with 30 in eBook format, 22 in Paperback format and 27 as Audio Books. I have an additional 12 books in development.

****

Books by Walter Parks

The Ancients:

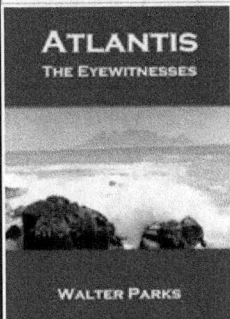

Atlantis the Eyewitnesses

A 9619 BC scroll proves that the Atlantis of Plato was real. We found Atlantis! See photos and artifacts.
See details.

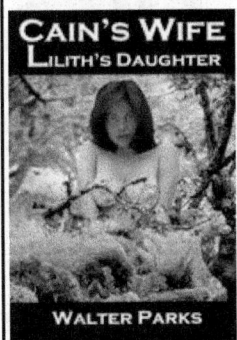

Cain's Wife, Lilith's Daughter

Evidence suggests Cain's wife was the daughter of Lilith; Adam's first wife. See the evidence.
See details.

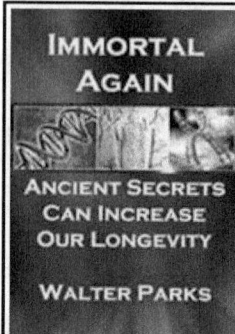

Immortal Again

Ancient Secrets Can Increase Our Longevity

We have used secrets from the ancients to make human cells immortal in the laboratory.

See details.

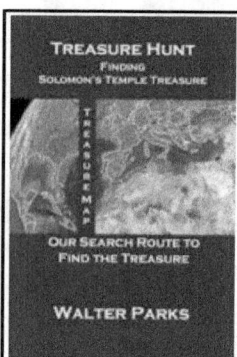

Treasure Hunt

Finding Solomon's Temple Treasure

We found Solomon's Temple Treasure after lost of 2000 years; worth a billion dollars.

See details.

Books by Walter Parks

Psychics & Unworldly:

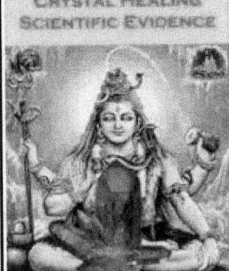

Crystal Healing Scientific Evidence
Crystal Healing evolved as our Third Eye evolved.
See details.

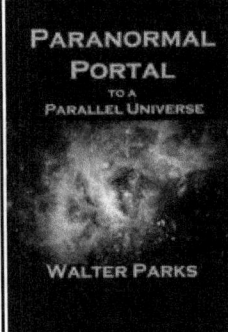

Paranormal Portal to a Parallel Universe
Our souls survive death in a parallel universe; key to the paranormal.
See details.

Books by Walter Parks

Creatism/Evolution:

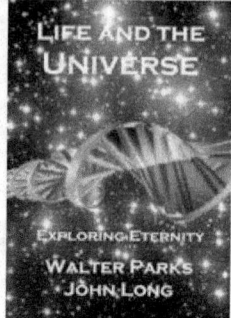

Life and the Universe
Exploring Eternity
See what we really know about life, about God, Parallel Universes and aliens.
See details.

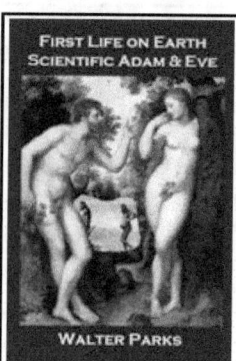

First Life on Earth
Scientific Adam & Eve
We share 90% of our DNA with cats, 80% with cows, 75% with mice, 60% with fruit fly, and 50% with the banana.
See details.

Books by Walter Parks

Anti-Aging and Health:

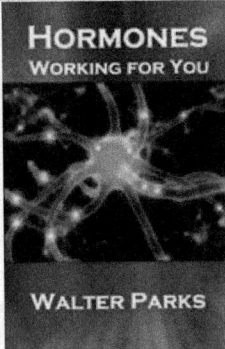

Hormones Working for You
Hormones regulate our bodies but they decline with age. Actions are needed to keep them healthy.
See details.

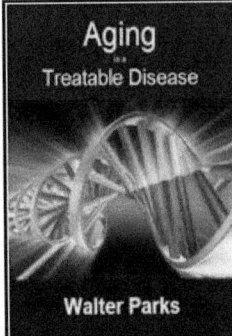

Aging is a Treatable Disease
Deterioration of the body that comes with growing old is not inevitable; aging is a treatable disease.
See details.

Books by Walter Parks

Military and Wars:

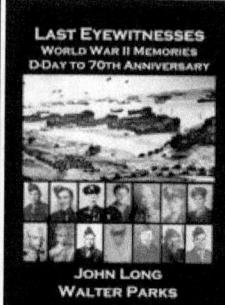

Last Eyewitnesses
World War II Memories D-Day to 70th Anniversary
World War II D-Day Memories; horrific images; bodies
stacked like cord wood; 4 feet high on the beach. We must
remember them!
See details.

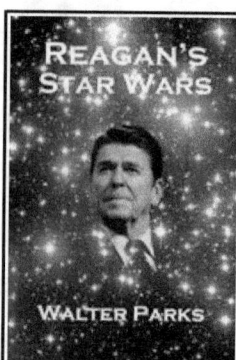

Reagan's Star Wars
The Military Industrial Complex
The military industrial complex used 3 basic fears to
leapfrog technology and create Reagan's Star Wars.
See details.

Books by Walter Parks

Religious Views:

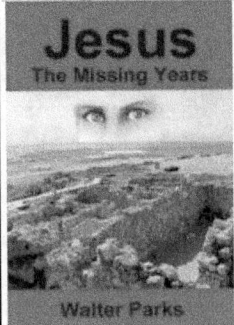

Jesus the Missing Years
Jesus was secluded in desert preparing for His ministry during His missing years; we have the scientific proof.
See details.

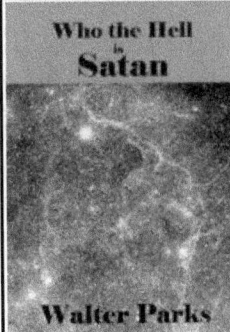

Who the Hell is Satan
The Bible tells us Satan was thrown from heaven. We found scientific proof of how and why.
See details.

Books by Walter Parks

Religious Views:

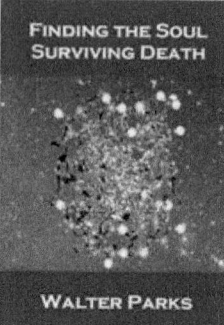

Finding the Soul
Surviving Death
We know we are going to die; we need a soul to have an afterlife. We may have found the scientific basis for the Soul.
See details.

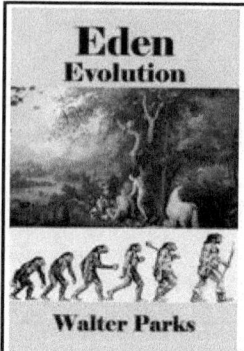

Eden Evolution
The Bible says God created Adam and Eve; science says we evolved from lower animals. See how both are correct.
See details.

Books by Walter Parks

Religious Views:

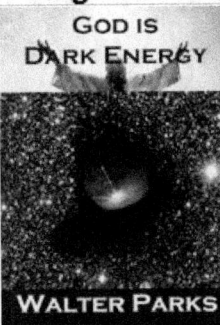

God is Dark Energy
Learn how God created the heavens and the earth; God is Dark Energy.
See details.

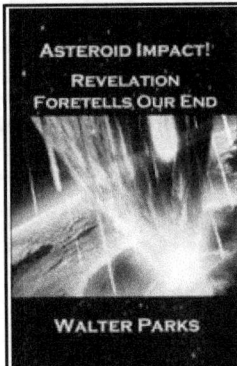

Asteroid Impact!
Revelation Foretells Our End
The Bible and scientific evidence tells us that we will be destroyed by an asteroid.
See details.

Books by Walter Parks

Almost True Stories:

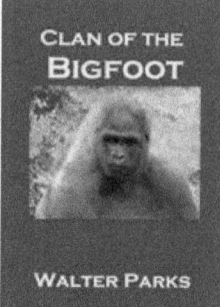

Clan of the Bigfoot
Early on we co-existed with 6 species of pre-humans; then just with Neanderthal. Now we've found bones showing that the Hobbit lived long after Neanderthal. Bigfoot is the next to be found.
See details.

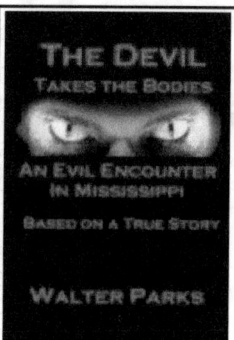

The Devil Takes the Bodies
An Evil Encounter in Mississippi
Based on a true story
The Devil is seen taking the bodies of dead women and girls just before their burial.
See details.

Books by Walter Parks

Almost True Stories:

Alligator Attack

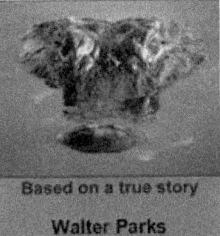

Based on a true story

Walter Parks

Alligator Attack!
Based on a true story
The Alligator got old Tom and then came for us.
See details.

Books in Development; Coming Soon:

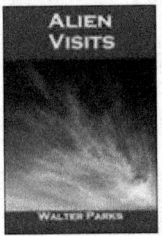

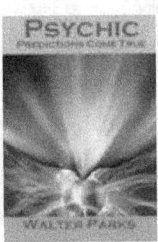

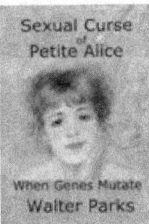

About
UnKnownTruths
Publishing Company

UnKnownTruths Publishing Company was formed to publish true stories of the unusual or of the previously Unknown or unexplained. These stories typically provide radically different views from those that have shaped the understandings of our natural world, our religions, our science, our history, and even the foundations of our civilizations.

The Company's stories also include stories of the very important anti-aging, life-extending medical breakthroughs; stem cell therapies; genetic therapies; cloning and other emerging findings that promise to change the very meaning of life.

The Company also publishes stories from the past that are so unbelievable that they are generally considered to be myths. The published stories provide the evidence for the truth.

The Company currently has an additional 12 books in development.

www.ingramcontent.com/pod-product-compliance
Lightning Source LLC
Chambersburg PA
CBHW062055280526
45788CB00003B/1240

* 9 7 8 1 4 6 0 9 6 1 9 3 3 *